KETO

MEAL PREP

*Lose Weight and Keep a Good Physical Form
with an Appropriate Nutrition*

MAX LOREN

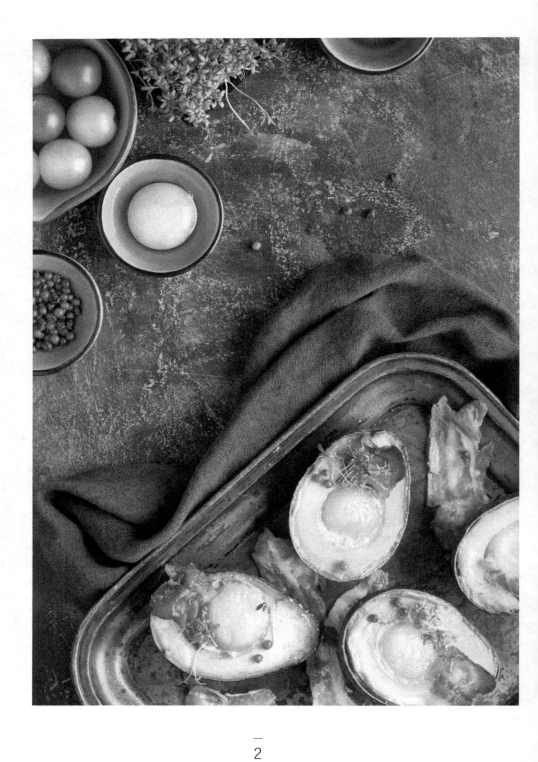

Legal Notice:

Disclaimer Notice:

Table of Contents

Sommario

Introduction

The ketogenic diet, or keto diet, is a low-carbohydrate, high-fat diet that provides many health benefits.Many studies have shown that this type of diet can help you reduce and improve your health.Ketogenic diets may even have benefits against diabetes, cancer, epilepsy, and Alzheimer's disease.

What is a ketogenic diet?

The ketogenic diet is a low carbohydrate, high-fat diet that has many similarities to the Atkins and low carb diets.It involves drastically reducing carbohydrate intake and replacing carbohydrates with fat. This drastic reduction in carbs puts your body into a metabolic state called ketosis.When this occurs, your body is incredibly efficient at burning fat for energy. It also converts fat into ketones within the liver, which can form the energy for the brain.Ketogenic diets can cause major reductions in blood glucose and insulin levels. This, along with the increase in ketones, has health benefits.

Different types of ketogenic diets

There are several versions of the ketogenic diet, including:

The standard ketogenic diet (SKD): This is often a low carb, moderate protein, and high-fat diet. It typically contains 70% fat, 20% protein, and only 10% carbs (9Trusted Source).

The cyclical ketogenic diet (CKD): This diet involves periods of upper carb refeeds, like 5 ketogenic days followed by 2 high carb days.

The targeted ketogenic diet (TKD): This diet allows you to feature carbs around workouts.

High protein ketogenic diet: this is often almost like a typical ketogenic diet, but includes more protein. The ratio is usually 60% fat, 35% protein, and 5% carbs.

However, only the quality and high protein ketogenic diets are studied extensively. Cyclical or targeted ketogenic diets are more advanced methods and are primarily employed by bodybuilders or athletes.

What is ketosis?

Ketosis may be a metabolic state during which your body uses fat for fuel rather than carbs.

It occurs once you significantly reduce your consumption of carbohydrates, limiting your body's supply of glucose (sugar), which is that the main source of energy for the cells.

Following a ketogenic diet is that the best thanks to entering ketosis. Generally, this involves limiting carb consumption to around 20 to 50 grams per day and filling abreast of fats, like meat, fish, eggs, nuts, and healthy oils

It's also important to moderate your protein consumption, this is often because protein can be converted into glucose if consumed in high amounts, which can slow your transition into ketosis

Practicing intermittent fasting could also assist you to enter ketosis faster. There are many various sorts of intermittent fasting, but the foremost common method involves limiting food intake to around 8 hours per day and fasting for the remaining 16 hours

Blood, urine, and breath tests are available, which may help determine whether you've entered ketosis by measuring the number of ketones produced by your body.

Certain symptoms can also indicate that you've entered ketosis, including increased thirst, dry mouth, frequent urination, and decreased hunger or appetite

Ketogenic diets can help you lose weight

A ketogenic diet is also an effective solution for losing weight and decreasing risk factors for disease.

Research has shown that the ketogenic diet can be very effective for weight loss as a low-fat diet.

What's more, the diet is so rich that you can lose weight without needing to count calories or track your food intake.

An analysis of 13 studies revealed that following a low-carb ketogenic diet was slightly superior for long-term weight loss compared to a low-fat diet.

It also led to a reduction in diastolic blood pressure and triglyceride levels.

Other health benefits of keto

- The ketogenic diet originated as a method of treating neurological diseases such as epilepsy.
- Studies have now shown that this diet may have benefits for a wide variety of different health conditions:

- Heart disease. The ketogenic diet can help improve risk factors such as body fat, HDL (good) cholesterol levels, blood pressure, and blood sugar.

- Cancer. Diet is currently being explored as an adjunct treatment for cancer because it may help slow tumor growth.

- Alzheimer's disease. The keto diet may help reduce the symptoms of Alzheimer's disease and slow its progression.

- Epilepsy. Research has shown that the ketogenic diet can cause significant reductions in seizures in epileptic children.

- Parkinson's disease. Although more research is needed, one study found that the diet helped improve symptoms of Parkinson's disease.

- Polycystic ovary syndrome. The ketogenic diet may help reduce insulin levels, which may play a key role in polycystic ovary syndrome.

- Brain injury. Some research suggests that the diet may improve the outcomes of traumatic brain injuries.

However, keep in mind that research in many of these areas is far from conclusive.

Foods to avoid

Any food high in carbohydrates should be reduced.

Here is a list of foods that should be reduced or eliminated on a ketogenic diet:

sugary foods: soda, juice, smoothies, cake, ice cream, candy, etc.

grains or starches: wheat products, rice, pasta, cereals, etc.

fruits: all fruits, except small portions of berries such as strawberries

beans or legumes: peas, beans, lentils, chickpeas, etc.

root and tuber vegetables: potatoes, sweet potatoes, carrots, parsnips, etc.

low-fat or diet products: low-fat mayonnaise, salad dressings, and condiments

some condiments or sauces: barbecue sauce, honey mustard, teriyaki sauce, ketchup, etc.

unhealthy fats: processed vegetable oils, mayonnaise, etc.

alcohol: beer, wine, liquor, mixed drinks

sugar-free diet foods: sugar-free candy, syrups, puddings, sweeteners, desserts, etc.

Foods to eat

You should focus most of your meals on these foods:

meat: red meat, steak, ham, sausage, bacon, chicken, and turkey

fatty fish: salmon, trout, tuna, and mackerel

eggs: whole pastured eggs or omega-3s

butter and cream: grass-fed butter and heavy cream

cheese: non-processed cheeses such as cheddar, goat, cream, blue, or mozzarella cheese

nuts and seeds: almonds, walnuts, flaxseeds, pumpkin seeds, chia seeds, etc.

healthy oils: extra virgin olive oil, coconut oil, and avocado oil

avocado: whole avocado or freshly made guacamole

low carb vegetables: green vegetables, tomatoes, onions, peppers, etc.

seasonings: salt, pepper, herbs, and spices

It's best to base your diet primarily on whole, single-ingredient foods. Here's a list of 44 healthy low-carb foods.

Healthy keto snacks

In case you get the urge to eat between meals, here are some healthy, keto-approved snacks:

fatty meat or fish

cheese

a handful of nuts or seeds

keto sushi bites

olives

one or two hard-boiled or deviled eggs

keto-friendly snack bars

90 percent dark chocolate

whole Greek yogurt mixed with nut butter and cocoa powder

peppers and guacamole

strawberries and plain cottage cheese

celery with salsa and guacamole

beef jerky

smaller portions of leftover meals

fat bombs

Keto tips and tricks

Although starting the ketogenic diet can be difficult, there are several tips and tricks you can use to make it easier.

Start by familiarizing yourself with food labels and checking the grams of fat, carbohydrates, and fiber to determine how your favorite foods can fit into your diet.

Planning your meals can also be beneficial and can help you save extra time during the week.

Tips for eating out on a ketogenic diet

Many restaurant meals can be made keto-friendly.

Most restaurants offer some type of meat or fish dish. Order this food and replace any high-carb food with extra vegetables.

Egg meals are also a good option, such as an omelet or eggs and bacon.

Another favorite meal is burgers without a bun. You could also replace the fries with veggies. Add extra avocado, cheese, bacon, or eggs.

In Mexican restaurants, you can enjoy any type of meat with extra cheese, guacamole, salsa, and sour cream.

For dessert, ask for a tray of mixed cheeses or berries with cream.

At least, in the beginning, it's crucial to eat until you're full and avoid cutting calories too much. Usually, a ketogenic diet involves weight loss without intentional calorie restriction.

In this Keto cookbook, you can organize your Keto diet with the different dishes you'll find for meals throughout the day. Enjoy!

Breakfast

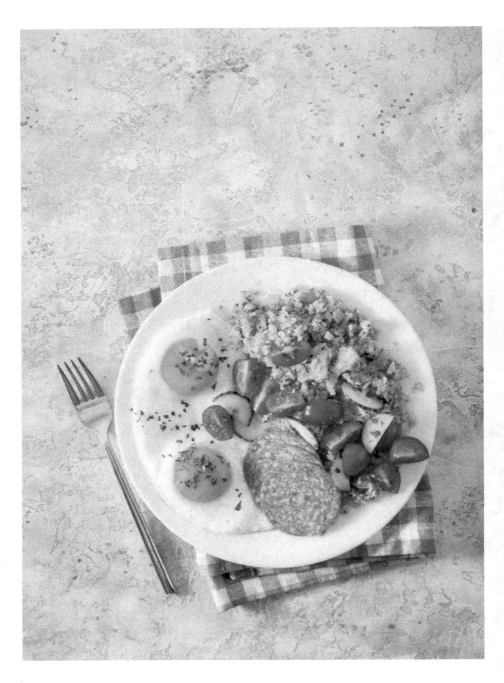

Colorful breakfast dish

Preparation time: 15 minutes
Cooking time: 8 hours
Servings: 12

Ingredients:
1/2 pound bulk crumbled Italian sausage
2 green onions
2 minced cloves garlic
1 chopped red bell pepper
18 eggs
1 cup almond milk
1 tsp. garlic powder
1 tsp. dried oregano
Black pepper

Directions:
Make sure to grease the slow cooker well before starting to use it.
Cook the Italian sausage first, with the green onions and garlic in a separate skillet for about 10-12 minutes. Drain the meat fat.
In the slow cooker, add the sausage, onions and garlic as well as the bell peppers.
In a separate bowl, combine the eggs, coconut milk, and all seasonings.
Cover the slow cooker and cook for about 6-8 hours. Serve warm.

Nutrition:
255 cal, 11.5 g total fat (3.6 g sat. fat), 172 mg chop. 119 mg sodium, 4.5 g carb. 4g fiber, 11.2g protein.

Egg Casserole

Preparation time: 2 hours
Servings: 4

Ingredients:
tomato, sliced
3 eggs
5 oz asparagus, chopped
4 oz Parmesan, chopped
1 oz fresh dill, chopped
1 teaspoon olive oil
¾ teaspoon salt
1 teaspoon paprika

Directions:
Mix up together olive oil, salt, paprika, chopped asparagus, and fresh dill.
Place the mixture in the slow cooker.
Add a layer of the sliced tomato.
Beat the eggs and pour over the tomatoes then close the lid.
Cook the casserole for 2 hours on High or until the eggs are solid.
Enjoy!

Nutrition:
calories 178, fat 11g, fiber 2.1g, carbs 7.5g, protein 15.7g

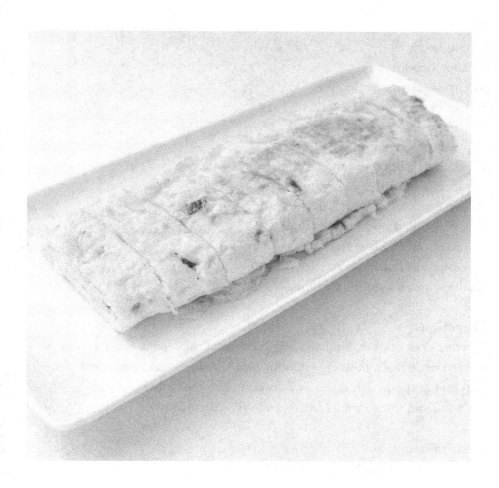

Coconut Raisins Oatmeal

Preparation time: 10 minutes
Cooking time: 8 hours
Servings: 2

Ingredients:
½ cup water
½ cup coconut milk
½ cup steel cut oats
½ cup carrots, grated
¼ cup raisins
A pinch of cinnamon powder
A pinch of ginger, ground
A pinch of nutmeg, ground
¼ cup coconut flakes, shredded
1 tablespoon orange zest, grated
½ teaspoon vanilla extract
½ tablespoon maple syrup
2 tablespoons walnuts, chopped

Directions:
In your slow cooker, mix water with coconut milk, oats, carrots, raisins, cinnamon, ginger, nutmeg, coconut flakes, orange zest, vanilla extract and maple syrup, stir, cover and cook on Low for 8 hours. Add walnuts, stir, divide into 2 bowls and serve for breakfast. Enjoy!

Nutrition:
calories 200, fat 4g, fiber 6g, carbs 8g, protein 8g

Green Shakshuka

Preparation Time: 15 minutes
Cooking Time: 10 minutes
Servings: 4

Ingredients:
tbsp. olive oil
tbsp. almond oil
1/2 medium green bell pepper, deseeded and chopped
1 celery stalk, chopped
1/4 cup (57 g) green beans, chopped
garlic clove, minced
tbsp. fresh mint leaves
tbsp. fresh parsley leaves
1/2 cup (113 g) baby kale
1/4 tsp. plain vinegar
Salt and black pepper to taste
1/4 tsp. nutmeg powder
7 oz. (200 g) feta cheese, divided
4 eggs

Directions:

Heat the olive oil and almond oil in a medium frying pan over medium heat. Add the bell pepper, celery, green beans, and sauté for 5 minutes or until the vegetables soften. Stir in the garlic, mint leaves, two tablespoons of parsley, and cook until fragrant, 1 minute. Add the kale, vinegar, and mix. Once the kale starts wilting, season with salt, black pepper, nutmeg powder, and stir in half of the feta cheese—Cook for 1 to 2 minutes. After, use the spatula to create four holes in the food and crack an egg into each hole. Cook until the egg whites set still running. Season the eggs with salt and black pepper. Turn the heat off and scatter the remaining feta cheese on top. Garnish with the remaining parsley and serve the shakshuka immediately.

Nutrition:

calories 322, fat 14.1g, fiber 10.3g, carbohydrates 9.4 g, protein 13.1g

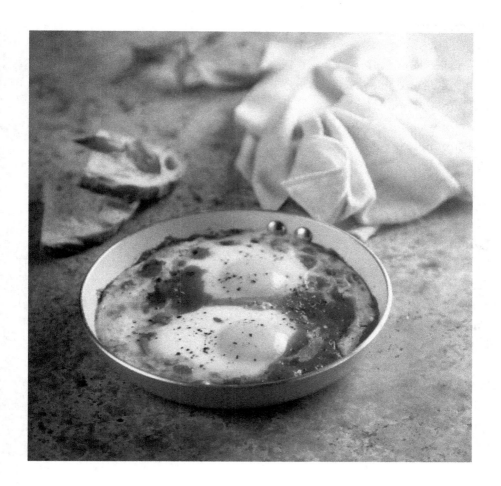

Coco-Nut" Granola

Preparation Time: 10 minutes
Cooking Time: 60 minutes
Servings: 8

Ingredients:
2 cups shredded unsweetened coconut
1 cup sliced almonds
1 cup raw sunflower seeds
1/2 cup raw pumpkin seeds
1/2 cup walnuts
1/2 cup melted coconut oil
10 drops liquid stevia
1 teaspoon ground cinnamon
1/2 teaspoon ground nutmeg

Directions:
Preheat the oven to 250°F. Line 2 baking sheets with parchment paper.
Set aside.
Toss all the ingredients together.
The granola will then put into baking sheets and spread it out evenly.
Bake the granola for about 1 hr.

Nutrition:
calories 131, fat 4.1g, fiber 5.8g, carbohydrates 2.8g, protein 5.6g

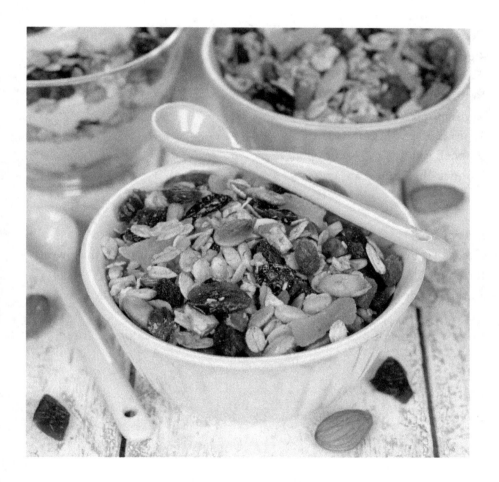

Cauliflower with Eggs

Preparation time: 10 minutes
Cooking time: 7 hours
Servings: 2

Ingredients:
Cooking spray
4 eggs, whisked
A pinch of salt and black pepper
¼ teaspoon thyme, dried
½ teaspoon turmeric powder
1 cup cauliflower florets
½ small yellow onion, chopped
3 ounces breakfast sausages, sliced
½ cup cheddar cheese, shredded

Directions:
Grease your slow cooker with cooking spray and spread the cauliflower florets on the bottom of the pot.
Add the eggs mixed with salt, pepper and the other ingredients and toss.
Put the lid on, cook on Low for 7 hours, divide between plates and serve for breakfast.

Nutrition:
calories 261, fat 6g, fiber 7g, carbs 22g, protein 6g

Bacon Artichoke Omelet

Preparation Time: 10 minutes
Cooking Time: 10 minutes
Servings: 4

Ingredients:
6 eggs, beaten
2 tablespoons heavy (whipping) cream
8 bacon slices, cooked and chopped
1 tablespoon olive oil
1/4 cup chopped onion
1/2 cup chopped artichoke hearts (canned, packed in water)
Sea salt
Freshly ground black pepper

Directions:
In a bowl or container, the eggs, heavy cream, and bacon must be mixed. Heat olive oil then sauté the onion until tender, about 3 minutes. Pour the egg mixture into the skillet for 1 minute. Cook the omelet, lifting the edges with a spatula to let the uncooked egg flow underneath, for 2 minutes. Sprinkle the artichoke hearts on top and flip the omelet. Cook for 4 minutes more until the egg is firm. Flip the omelet over again, so the artichoke hearts are on top. Remove from the heat, cut the omelet into quarters, and season with salt and black pepper. Transfer the omelet to plates and serve.

Nutrition:
calories 314, fat 7.1g, fiber 5.4g, carbohydrates 3.1g, protein 8.5g

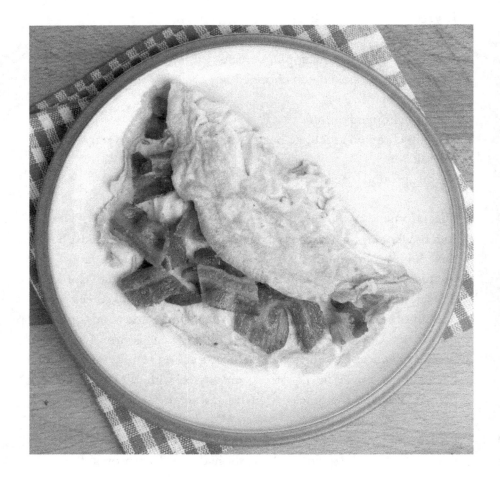

Chicken

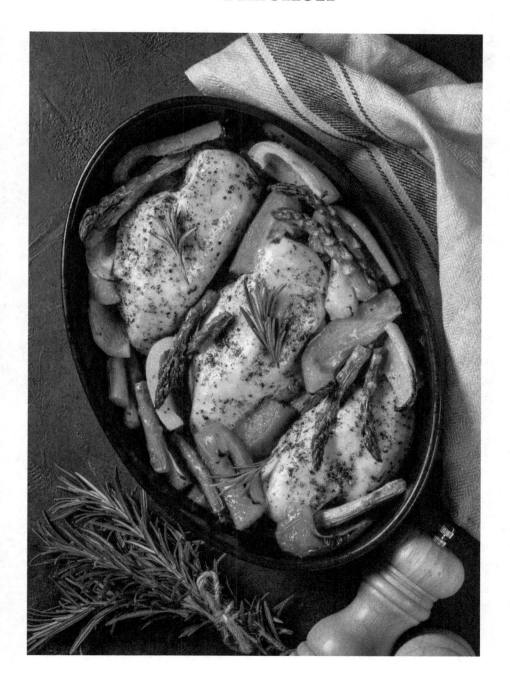

Chicken with Cream of Mushroom Soup

Preparation time: 10 minutes
Cooking time: 15 minutes
Servings: 2

Ingredients:
1 tablespoon olive oil
yellow onion, chopped
garlic cloves, pressed
2 chicken breast, skinless and boneless, cut into bite-sized pieces
½ cup cream of mushroom soup

Directions:
Heat the olive oil in a saucepan over medium-high heat. Once hot, sweat the yellow onion until tender and translucent about 3 minutes. Then, cook the garlic until aromatic or about 30 seconds.

Then, sear the chicken breast for 3 minutes, stirring frequently to ensure even cooking. Pour in the cream of mushroom soup and stir to combine.

Turn the heat to medium-low and let it simmer until the sauce has reduced by half or 6 to 8 minutes longer. Serve immediately.

Nutrition:
calories 336, fat 20.7g, protein 30.7g, carbs 4.2g, net carbs 3.7g, fiber 0.5g

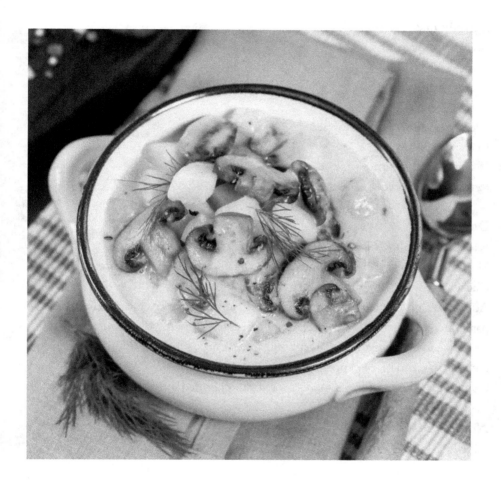

Chicken and Broccoli Marsala

Preparation time: 10 minutes
Cooking time: 15 minutes
Servings: 2

Ingredients:
tablespoon olive oil
chicken fillets
¼ cup marsala wine
1 cup broccoli florets
1 teaspoon fresh garlic, chopped
¼ tomato paste
½ cup double cream
½ teaspoon paprika

Directions:
Sea salt and ground black pepper, to taste
Heat the olive oil in a frying pan over a moderate flame. Once hot, brown the chicken fillets for 7 minutes on each side.
Add a splash of wine to deglaze the pot. Add in the broccoli, garlic, and tomato paste and gently stir to combine. Turn the heat to simmer.
Continue to cook an additional 5 minutes. After that, stir in the double cream, paprika, salt, and black pepper.
Continue to simmer for 5 minutes more or until heated through. Bon appétit!

Nutrition:
calories 350, fat 20.5g, protein 35.2g, carbs 4.6g, net carbs 3.4g, fiber 1.2g

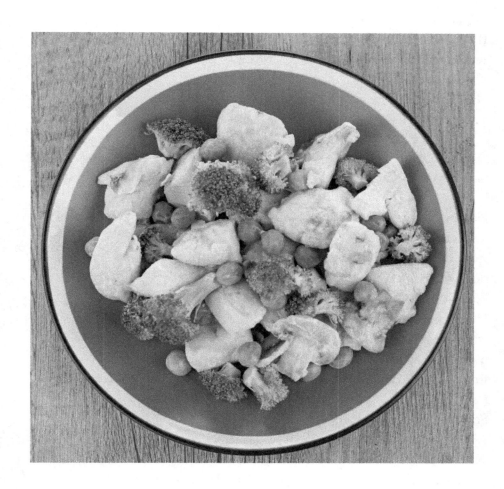

Rice Wine Duck with White Onion

Preparation time: 5 minutes
Cooking time: 25 minutes
Servings: 6

Ingredients:

1½ pounds (680 g) duck breast
1 tablespoon sesame oil
1 white onion, chopped
¼ cup rice wine
3 teaspoons soy sauce

Directions:

Gently score the duck breast skin in a tight crosshatch pattern using a sharp knife.

Heat the sesame oil in a skillet over moderate heat. Now, sauté the onion until tender and translucent.

Add in the duck breasts; sear the duck breasts for 10 to 13 minutes or until the skin looks crispy with golden brown color; drain off the duck fat from the skillet.

Flip the breasts over and sear the other side for 3 minutes. Deglaze the skillet with rice wine, scraping up any brown bits stuck to the bottom. Transfer to a baking pan; add the rice wine and soy sauce to the baking pan.

Roast in the preheated oven at 400°F (205°C) for 4 minutes for medium-rare (145°F / 63°C), or 6 minutes for medium (165°F / 74°C).

Serve garnished with sesame seeds if desired. Enjoy!

Nutrition:

calories 264, fat 11.4g, protein 34.2g, carbs 3.6g, net carbs 3.0g, fiber 0.6g

Whole Chicken with Leek and Mushrooms

Preparation time: 15 minutes
Cooking time: 45 minutes
Servings: 4

Ingredients:
tablespoon olive oil
1½ pounds (680 g) whole chicken, skinless and boneless
cups button mushrooms, sliced
1 serrano pepper, sliced
1 medium-sized leek, chopped
teaspoon ginger-garlic paste
¼ cup dry red wine
Sea salt and ground black pepper, to season
tablespoons capers
1 cup tomato paste

Directions:
Heat the olive oil in a frying pan over a moderate flame. Fry the
chicken until golden brown on all sides or about 10 minutes; set aside.
Then, cook the mushrooms, serrano pepper, and leek in the pan
drippings. Cook until they have softened or about 6 minutes.
After that, stir in the ginger-garlic paste and fry for a further 30
seconds. Add a splash of red wine to deglaze the pan.
Add the chicken back to the frying pan. Add in salt, black pepper,
capers, and tomato paste; stir to combine well and bring to a rapid boil.
Turn the heat to medium-low and let it cook for 30 minutes more or
until everything is heated through. Serve immediately.

Nutrition:
calories 425, fat 29.1g, protein 33.4g, carbs 5.6g, net carbs 4.4g,
fiber 1.2g

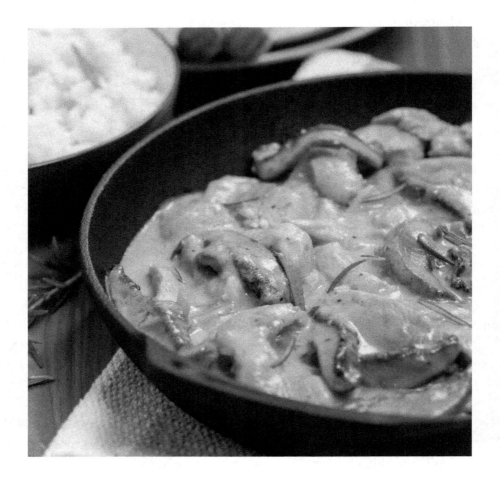

Buffalo Chicken Bake

Preparation time: 10 minutes
Cooking time: 55 minutes
Servings: 6

Ingredients:
tablespoon olive oil
pounds (907 g) chicken drumettes
Sauce:
½ cup melted butter
½ cup hot sauce
2 tablespoons white vinegar
¼ teaspoon granulated garlic
Sea salt and ground black, to season

Directions:
Start by preheating your oven to 320°F (160°C). Brush a baking pan with olive oil. Arrange the chicken drumettes in the greased pan.
Prepare the sauce by whisking the melted butter, hot sauce, white vinegar, garlic, salt and black pepper until well combined.
Pour the sauce over the chicken drumettes. Bake for 55 minutes, flipping the chicken drumettes once or twice.
Taste, adjust the seasonings and serve warm.

Nutrition:
calories 289, fat 20.5g, protein 23.4g, carbs 1.3g, net carbs 1.0g, fiber 0.3g

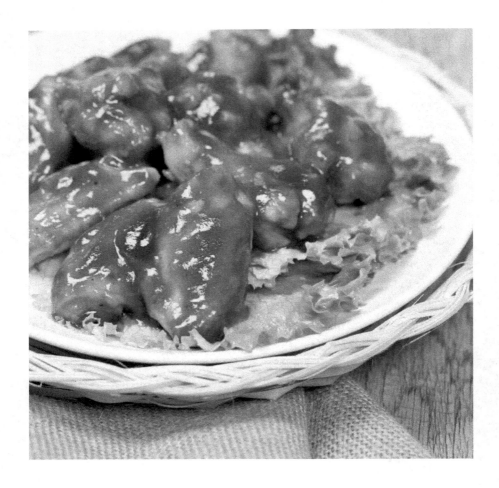

Whole Chicken with Leek and Mushrooms

Preparation time: 15 minutes
Cooking time: 45 minutes
Servings: 4

Ingredients:
tablespoon olive oil
1½ pounds (680 g) whole chicken, skinless and boneless
cups button mushrooms, sliced
1 serrano pepper, sliced
1 medium-sized leek, chopped
teaspoon ginger-garlic paste
¼ cup dry red wine
Sea salt and ground black pepper, to season
tablespoons capers
1 cup tomato paste

Directions:
Heat the olive oil in a frying pan over a moderate flame. Fry the chicken until golden brown on all sides or about 10 minutes; set aside. Then, cook the mushrooms, serrano pepper, and leek in the pan drippings. Cook until they have softened or about 6 minutes. After that, stir in the ginger-garlic paste and fry for a further 30 seconds. Add a splash of red wine to deglaze the pan. Add the chicken back to the frying pan. Add in salt, black pepper, capers, and tomato paste; stir to combine well and bring to a rapid boil. Turn the heat to medium-low and let it cook for 30 minutes more or until everything is heated through. Serve immediately.

Nutrition:
calories 425, fat 29.1g, protein 33.4g, carbs 5.6g, net carbs 4.4g, fiber 1.2g

Chicken Pot Pie

Preparation Time: 15 minutes
Cooking Time: 25 minutes
Servings: 4

Ingredients:
For the filling
1/2 medium onion, chopped
2 celery stalks, chopped
1/2 cup fresh or frozen peas
2 tablespoons butter
1 garlic clove, minced
11/2 pounds chicken thighs
1 cup chicken broth
1/2 cup heavy (whipping) cream
1/2 cup shredded low-moisture mozzarella cheese
1 teaspoon dried thyme
1/2 teaspoon pink Himalayan sea salt
1/2 teaspoon freshly ground black pepper
For the crust
cup almond flour
tablespoons butter, at room temperature
2 tablespoons sour cream
1 large egg white
1 tablespoon ground flaxseed
1 teaspoon xanthan gum
1 teaspoon baking powder
1/2 teaspoon garlic powder
1/4 teaspoon pink Himalayan sea salt
1/4 teaspoon dried thyme

Directions:

Filling: In a saucepan, combine the onion, celery, peas, butter, and garlic over medium heat. Cook for about 5 minutes, until the onion starts to turn translucent. In a large skillet, cook the chicken thighs for 3 to 5 minutes, until there is no more visible pink. Add the cooked chicken and all juices to the pan with the vegetables. Add the broth, cream, mozzarella, thyme, salt, and pepper to the pan. Simmer it until sauce thickens, stirring occasionally. Preheat the oven to 400°F. In a bowl or container, combine the almond flour, butter, sour cream, egg white, flaxseed, xanthan gum, baking powder, garlic powder, salt, and thyme. Form this into a dough. Place the dough between 2 sheets of parchment paper and roll out into a 10-inch round that is 1/4 inch thick. Fill an 8-inch pie pan or 4 (6-ounce) ramekins with the chicken filling. Top the pie pan with the crust, flipping it onto the filling and peeling away the parchment paper. If using ramekins, cut circles of the dough and fit them onto the ramekins. Pinch to seal the edges, and trim off any excess.

Baking time: 10-12 minutes Let cool for 5 minutes, then serve.

Nutrition:

calories 341, fat 18.4g, fiber 10.3g, carbohydrates 4.1 g, p12.5g

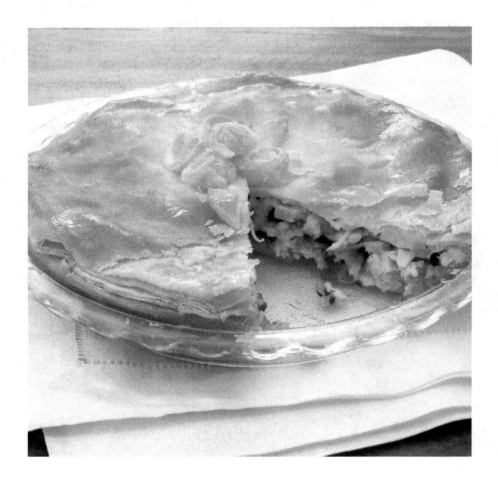

Pork

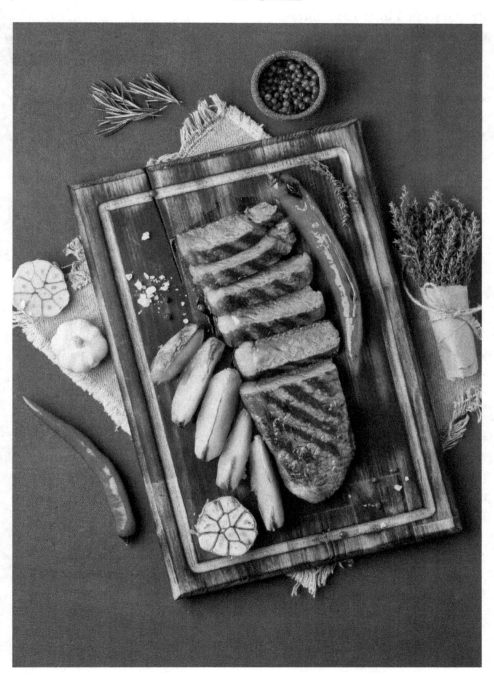

Ground Beef Stroganoff

Preparation Time: 10 minutes
Cooking Time: 15 minutes
Servings: 4

Ingredients:
2 tbsp. butter
1 clove minced garlic
1 pound 80% lean ground beef
Salt and pepper, to taste
10 oz(228g) sliced mushrooms
2 tbsp. water
1 cup sour cream
1 tbsp. fresh lemon juice
1 tbsp. fresh chopped parsley

Directions:
The butter must be added to a pan. When the butter has melted and stops foaming, add the minced garlic to the skillet. Cook the garlic until fragrant, then mix in the ground beef—season with salt and pepper. Cook the ground beef until no longer pink; break up the grounds with a wooden spoon. Add the water and mushrooms to the pan and cook over medium heat. Cook until the liquid has reduced halfway, and the mushrooms are tender. Set the cooked mushrooms aside. Reduce the heat, then whisk the sour cream and paprika into the skillet. Stir in the cooked beef and mushrooms into the pan and combine. Stir in the lemon juice and parsley.

Nutrition:
calories 380, fat 5.1g, fiber 3.6g, carbohydrates 12.3 g, protein 15.4g

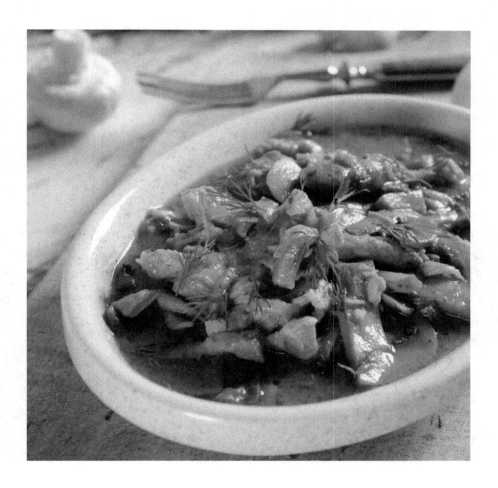

Pulled Boston Butt

Preparation time: 15 minutes
Cooking time: 5 minutes
Servings: 2

Ingredients:
teaspoon lard, melted at room temperature
¾ pork Boston butt, sliced
garlic cloves, pressed
½ teaspoon red pepper flakes, crushed
½ teaspoon black peppercorns, freshly cracked
Sea salt, to taste
2 bell peppers, deveined and sliced
1 tablespoon fresh mint leaves, snipped
4 tablespoons cream cheese

Directions:
Melt the lard in a cast-iron skillet over a moderate flame. Once hot, brown the pork for 2 minutes per side until caramelized and crispy on the edges.
Reduce the temperature to medium-low and continue cooking another 4 minutes, turning over periodically. Shred the pork with two forks and return to the skillet.
Add the garlic, red pepper, black peppercorns, salt, and bell pepper and continue cooking for a further 2 minutes or until the peppers are just tender and fragrant.
Serve with fresh mint and a dollop of cream cheese. Enjoy!

Nutrition:
calories 371, fat 21.8g, protein 35.0g, carbs 5.0g, net carbs 4.0g, fiber 1.0g

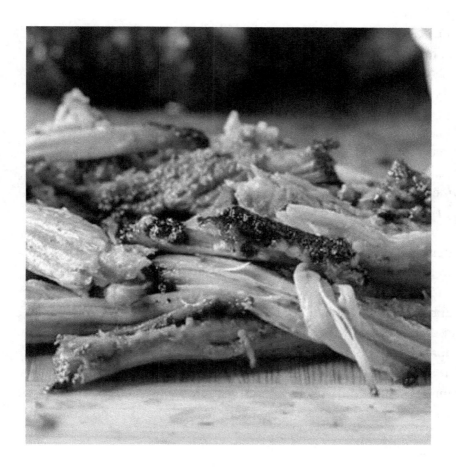

Pork Chops in Blue Cheese Sauce

Preparation Time: 5 minutes
Cooking Time: 10 minutes
Servings: 2

Ingredients:
2 boneless pork chops
Pink Himalayan salt
Freshly ground black pepper
2 tablespoons butter
1/3 cup blue cheese crumbles
1/3 cup heavy (whipping) cream
1/3 cup sour cream

Directions:
Dry the pork chops and season with pink Himalayan salt and pepper.
In a medium skillet over medium heat, melt the butter. When the
butter melts and is very hot, add the pork chops and sear on each side
for 3 minutes. The pork chops must be transferred to a plate and let
rest for 3 to 5 minutes. In a preheated pan, melt the blue cheese
crumbles, frequently stirring so they don't burn. Add the cream and the
sour cream to the pan with the blue cheese. Let simmer for a few
minutes, stirring occasionally. For an extra kick of flavor in the sauce,
pour the pork-chop pan juice into the cheese mixture and stir. Let
simmer while the pork chops are resting. Put the pork chops on two
plates, pour the blue cheese sauce over the top of each, and serve.

Nutrition:
calories 434, fat 14.1g, fiber 11.3g, carbohydrates 3.1g, protein 17.5g

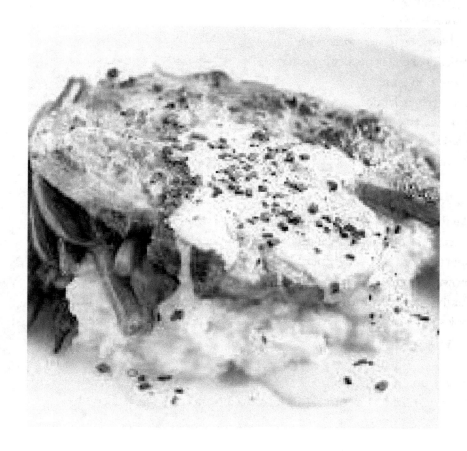

Pork and Cucumber Lettuce Cups

Preparation time: 10 minutes
Cooking time: 15 minutes
Servings: 6

Ingredients:
2 pounds (907 g) ground pork
1 tablespoon ginger- garlic paste
Pink salt and chili pepper to taste
1 teaspoon butter
head Iceberg lettuce
sprigs green onion, chopped
1 red bell pepper, seeded and chopped
½ cucumber, finely chopped

Directions:
Put the pork with ginger-garlic paste, salt, and chili pepper seasoning in a saucepan. Cook for 10 minutes over medium heat while breaking any lumps until the pork is no longer pink. Drain liquid and add the butter, melt and brown the meat for 4 minutes, continuously stirring. Turn the heat off.
Pat the lettuce dry with a paper towel and in each leaf, spoon two to three tablespoons of pork, top with green onions, bell pepper, and cucumber. Serve with soy drizzling sauce.

Nutrition:
calories 312, fat 24.2g, protein 19.1g, carbs 3.1g, net carbs 1.0g, fiber 2.1g

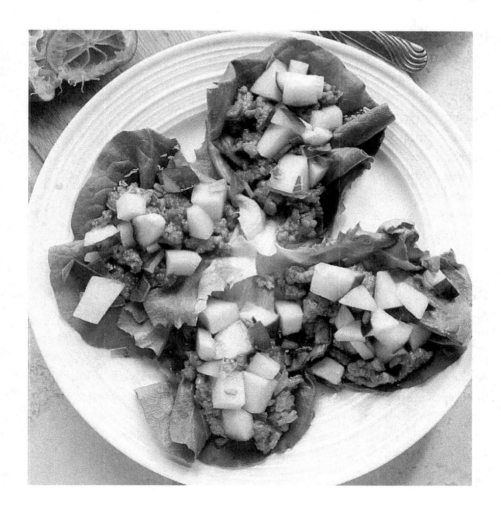

Creamy Pepper Loin Steaks

Preparation time: 15 minutes
Cooking time: 10 minutes
Servings: 2

Ingredients:
teaspoon lard, at room temperature
pork loin steaks
½ cup beef bone broth
2 bell peppers, deseeded and chopped
1 shallot, chopped
1 garlic clove, minced
Sea salt, to season
½ teaspoon cayenne pepper
¼ teaspoon paprika
1 teaspoon Italian seasoning mix
¼ cup Greek yogurt

Directions:
Melt the lard in a cast-iron skillet over moderate heat. Once hot, cook the pork loin steaks until slightly browned or approximately 5 minutes per side; reserve.

Add a splash of the beef bone broth to deglaze the pan. Now, cook the bell peppers, shallot, and garlic until tender and aromatic. Season with salt, cayenne pepper, paprika, and Italian seasoning mix.

After that, decrease the temperature to medium-low, add the Greek yogurt to the skillet and let it simmer for 2 minutes more or until heated through. Serve immediately.

Nutrition:
calories 450, fat 19.1g, protein 62.2g, carbs 6.0g, net carbs 4.9g, fiber 1.1g

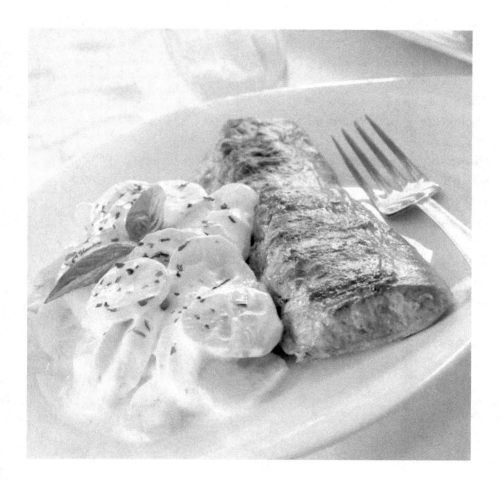

Pork Medallions with Onions and Bacon

Preparation time: 10 minutes
Cooking time: 25 minutes
Servings: 4

Ingredients:
2 onions, chopped
6 bacon slices, chopped
½ cup vegetable stock
Salt and black pepper, to taste
1 pound (454 g) pork tenderloin, cut into medallions

Directions:
Set a pan over medium heat, stir in the bacon, cook until crispy, and remove to a plate. Add onions, black pepper, and salt, and cook for 5 minutes; set to the same plate with bacon.
Add the pork medallions to the pan, season with black pepper and salt, brown for 3 minutes on each side, turn, reduce heat to medium, and cook for 7 minutes. Stir in the stock, and cook for 2 minutes. Return the bacon and onions to the pan and cook for 1 minute.

Nutrition:
calories 326, fat 17.9g, protein 35.9g, carbs 7.2g, net carbs 5.9g, fiber 1.3g

Mediterranean Spiced Pork Roast

Preparation time: 10 minutes
Cooking time: 3 hours 50 minutes
Servings: 4

Ingredients:
2 pounds (907 g) pork shoulder
2 tablespoons coconut aminos
½ cup red wine
1 tablespoon Dijon mustard
1 tablespoon Mediterranean spice mix

Directions:
Place the pork shoulder, coconut aminos, wine, mustard, and Mediterranean spice mix in a ceramic dish.
Cover and let it marinate in your refrigerator for 2 hours. Meanwhile, preheat your oven to 420°F (216°C).
Place the pork shoulder on a rack set into a roasting pan. Roast for 15 to 20 minutes; reduce the heat to 330°F (166°C).
Roast an additional 3 hours and 30 minutes, basting with the reserved marinade. Bon appétit!

Nutrition:
calories 610, fat 40.2g, protein 57.0g, carbs 0.7g, net carbs 0.6g, fiber 0.1g

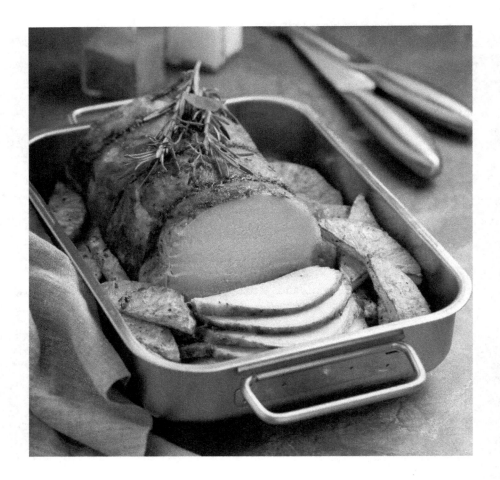

Fish and Seafood

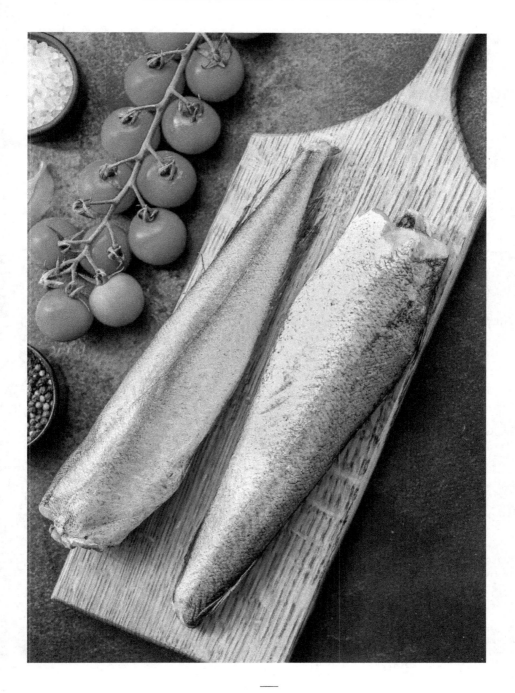

Cardamom Trout

Preparation time: 10 minutes
Cooking time: 2.5 hours
Servings: 4

Ingredients:
1 teaspoon ground cardamom
1-pound trout fillet
1 teaspoon butter, melted
1 tablespoon lemon juice
¼ cup of water
1.2 teaspoon salt

Directions:
In the shallow bowl mix butter, lemon juice, and salt.
Then sprinkle the trout fillet with ground cardamom and butter mixture.
Place the fish in the slow cooker and add water.
Cook the meal on High for 2.5 hours.

Nutrition:
226 calories, 30.3g protein, 0.4g carbohydrates, 10.6g fat, 0.2g fiber, 86mg cholesterol, 782mg sodium, 536mg potassium.

Creamy Bay Scallops

Preparation time: 10 minutes
Cooking time: 6 hours
Servings: 4

Ingredients:

¼ cup butter
1 tablespoon shallots, diced
¼ cup dry white wine
tablespoon lemon juice
cups mushrooms, quartered
¼ cup fresh parsley, chopped
½ cup heavy cream
¼ cup crème fraiche
1 teaspoon salt
1 teaspoon black pepper
1 pound bay scallops
½ cup Gruyere cheese, cubed

Directions:

Combine the butter, shallots, white wine, and lemon juice in a slow cooker.

Cover and cook on high for 2 hours. Remove the lid from the slow cooker and add the mushrooms, parsley, heavy cream, crème fraiche, salt, and black pepper. Mix well, cover, and cook for 5-10 minutes to bring the heat of the liquid back up. Add the scallops and Gruyere cheese. Cook an additional 30-35 minutes, or until the scallops are cooked through.

Nutrition:

Fat 32g, Carbs 5.6g, Protein 25.3g, Dietary Fiber 0.4g , Sugars 1.1g

Garlic Butter Tilapia with Orange

Preparation time: 10 minutes
Cooking time: 6 hours
Servings: 4

Ingredients:
4 tilapia fillets
4 minced garlic cloves, divided
4 tablespoons unsalted butter, softened and divided
1 10-ounce can mandarin oranges, drained
Salt and white pepper

Directions:
Prepare 4 sheets of aluminum foil to hold and cover each fillet.
Place the fish on the foil. Sprinkle some 1 minced garlic clove and top
with 1 tablespoon of butter. Top with ¼ of the mandarin oranges.
Sprinkle with salt and white pepper. Fold the foil over the fish to seal
in the flavors.
Do the same for the rest of the fillets.
Place in the slow cooker, cover and cook for 2 hours on HIGH, or
until the fish is cooked through.

Nutrition:
calories 154, fat 1g, carbs 4g, protein 14g, sodium 240mg

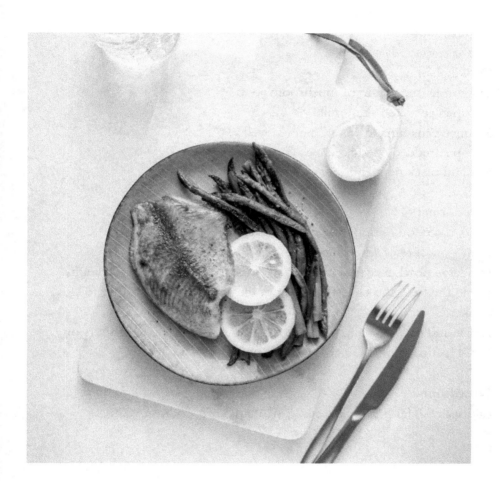

Classic Slow Cooked Tuna Noodle Casserole

Preparation time: 10 minutes
Cooking time: 4 hours
Servings: 6

Ingredients:
2 cups egg noodles
Cooking spray
can condensed cream of mushroom soup
½ cup evaporated skim milk
5-ounce cans tuna in water, drained well
½ cup shredded cheddar cheese
Salt and black pepper

Directions:
Cook the noodles until just a little underdone (al dente). Drain.
Coat slow cooker with nonstick cooking spray.
In a large bowl, mix the soup and milk until well blended and creamy.
Stir in the tuna and cheese. Stir in noodles and transfer mixture to slow cooker.
Cover and cook for 3 to 4 hours on LOW or for 1-1/2 to 2 hours on HIGH, stirring occasionally.

Nutrition:
calories 300, fat 5.3g, carbs 31.2g, protein 30.7g, sodium 922mg

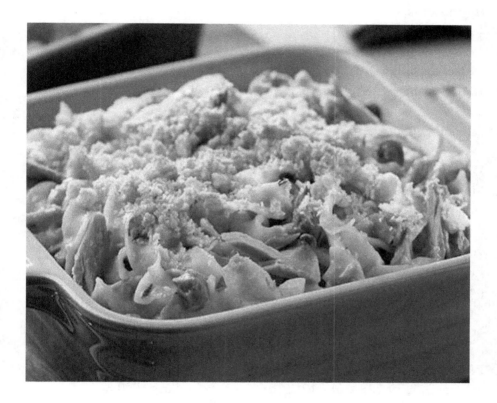

Buttery Salmon with Onions and Carrots

Preparation time: 10 minutes
Cooking time: 2 hours
Servings: 4

Ingredients:
4 salmon fillets
4 tablespoons butter
4 onions, chopped
16 ounces baby carrots
3 cloves garlic, minced
Salt and pepper

Directions:
Melt butter in the microwave, and pour into the slow cooker.
Add onions, garlic, and baby carrots.
Cover and cook for 6-7 hours on LOW, stirring occasionally until vegetables begin to caramelize.
Place fillet over vegetables in slow cooker, and season with salt and pepper.
Cover and cook on LOW for 1-2 hours until salmon flakes.
Serve on a serving plate, and top with onion mixture.

Nutrition:
calories 367, fat 22g, carbs 12.2g, protein 39g, sodium 1090mg

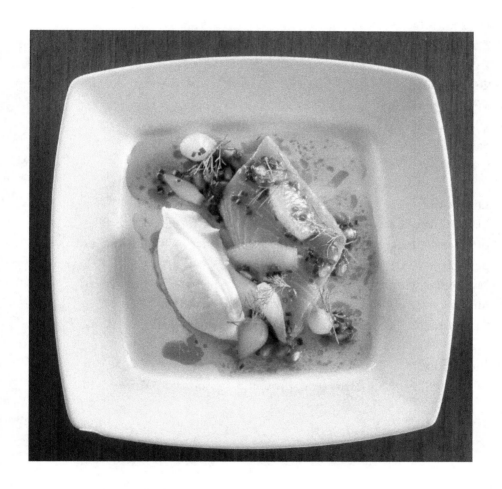

Garlic Butter Tilapia

Preparation time: 10 minutes
Cooking time: 6 hours
Servings: 4

Ingredients:
2 tablespoons butter, at room temperature
2 garlic cloves, minced
2 teaspoons flat parsley, chopped
4 tilapia fillets
1 lemon, cut into wedges
Salt and Pepper to taste
Cooking spray

Directions:
Place a large sheet of aluminum foil on a work surface. Place fillets in the middle. Place in a slow cooker. Season generously with salt and pepper.
Mix butter with minced garlic and chopped parsley. Evenly spread mixture over each fillet. Wrap foil around fish, sealing all sides.
Cook on HIGH for 2 hours. Serve with lemon wedges.

Nutrition:
calories 89, fat 9.8g, carbs 0.5g, protein 8.4g, sodium 202mg

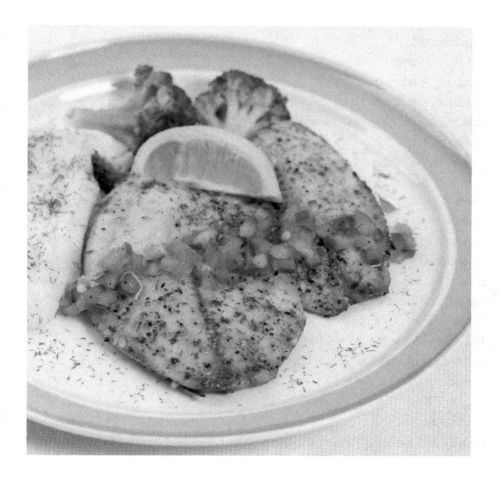

Sour Cream Salmon Steaks

Preparation time: 10 minutes
Cooking time: 20 minutes
Servings: 4

Ingredients:
1 cup sour cream
½ tablespoon minced dill
½ lemon, zested and juiced
Pink salt and black pepper to season
4 salmon steaks
½ cup grated Parmesan cheese

Directions:
Preheat oven to 400°F (205°C) and line a baking sheet with parchment paper; set aside. In a bowl, mix the sour cream, dill, lemon zest, juice, salt and black pepper, and set aside.

Season the fish with salt and black pepper, drizzle lemon juice on both sides of the fish and arrange them in the baking sheet. Spread the sour cream mixture on each fish and sprinkle with Parmesan.

Bake the fish for 15 minutes and after broil the top for 2 minutes with a close watch for a nice a brown color. Plate the fish and serve with buttery green beans.

Nutrition:
calories 289, fat 23.5g, protein 16.1g, carbs .5g, net carbs 1.3g, fiber 0.2g

Soup

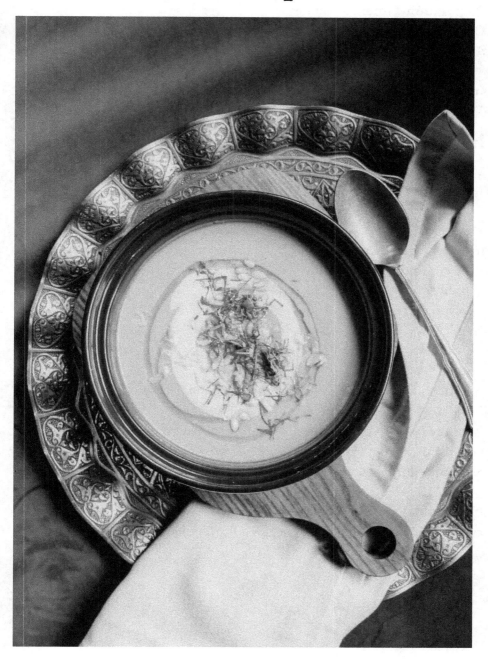

Hearty Fall Stew

Preparation Time: 15 minutes
Cooking Time: 8 hrs.
Servings: 6

Ingredients:
3 tablespoons extra-virgin olive oil, divided
1 (2-pound / 907-g) beef chuck roast, cut into 1-inch chunks
1/2 teaspoon salt
1/4 teaspoon freshly ground black pepper
1/4 cup apple cider vinegar
1/2 sweet onion, chopped
1 cup diced tomatoes
teaspoon dried thyme
11/2 cups pumpkin, cut into 1-inch chunks
cups beef broth
2 teaspoons minced garlic
1 tablespoon chopped fresh parsley, for garnish

Directions:
Add the beef to the skillet, and sprinkle salt and pepper to season.
Cook the beef for 7 minutes or until well browned.
Put the cooked beef into the slow cooker and add the remaining
ingredients, except for the parsley, to the slow cooker. Stir to mix well.
Slow cook for 8 hrs. and top with parsley before serving.

Nutrition:
calories 462, fat 19.1g, fiber 11.6g, carbohydrates 10.7g, protein 18.6g

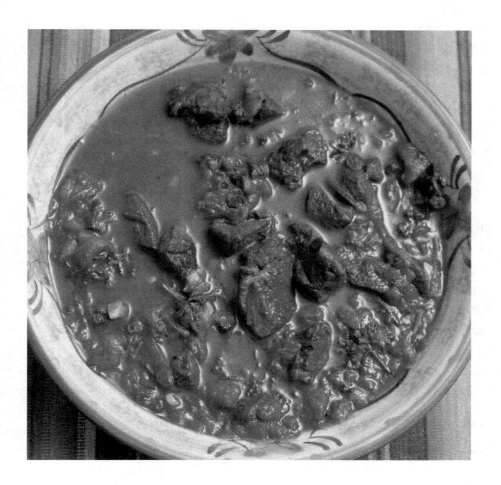

Creamy Asparagus Soup

Preparation Time: 10 minutes
Cooking Time: 15 minutes
Servings: 4

Ingredients:
2 lbs. asparagus, cut the ends and chop into 1/2-inch pieces
tbsp. olive oil
garlic cloves, minced
2 oz parmesan cheese, grated
1/2 cup heavy cream
1/4 cup onion, chopped
4 cups vegetable stock
Pepper
Salt

Directions:
Heat olive oil in a large pot over medium heat. Add onion to the pot and sauté until onion is softened. Add asparagus and sauté for 2-3 minutes. Add garlic and sauté for a minute. Season with pepper and salt. Add stock and bring to boil. Turn heat to low and simmer until asparagus is tender. Remove pot from heat and puree the soup using an immersion blender until creamy. Return pot on heat. Add cream and stir well and cook over medium heat until just soup is hot. Do not boil the soup. Remove from heat. Add cheese and stir well. Serve and enjoy.

Nutrition:
calories 202, fat 8.4g, fiber 6.1g, carbohydrates 3.1 g, protein 5.3g

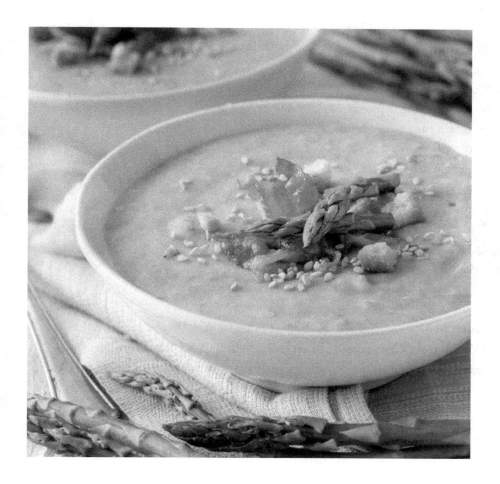

Clam Soup

Preparation time: 10 minutes
Cooking time: 1.5 hours
Servings: 2

Ingredients:
¼ teaspoon ground black pepper
¼ teaspoon chili flakes
3 cups fish stock
8 oz. clams, canned
oz. scallions, chopped
tablespoons sour cream
½ teaspoon dried thyme
Pour fish stock in the slow cooker.

Directions:
Add canned clams, chili flakes, ground black pepper, scallions, and dried thyme.
Add sour cream and dried thyme.
Cook the soup on High for 1.5 hours.

Nutrition:
145 calories, 9.3g protein, 14.3g carbohydrates, 5.6g fat, 1g fiber, 9mg cholesterol, 965mg sodium, 667mg potassium.

Bacon and Chicken Soup

Preparation time: 15 minutes
Cooking time: 8 hours
Servings: 8

Ingredients:
1 tablespoon extra-virgin olive oil
6 cups chicken broth
3 cups cooked chicken, chopped
sweet onion, chopped
celery stalks, chopped
carrot, diced
teaspoons minced garlic
1½ cups heavy whipping cream
1 cup cream cheese
1 cup cooked chopped bacon
1 tablespoon chopped fresh parsley, for garnish

Directions:
Lightly grease the insert of the slow cooker with the olive oil.
Add the broth, chicken, onion, celery, carrot, and garlic.
Cover and cook on low for 8 hours.
Stir in the heavy cream, cream cheese, and bacon.
Serve topped with the parsley.

Nutrition:
calories 489, fat 36.9g, protein 26.9g, carbs 10.9g, net carbs 9.8g, fiber 1.1g

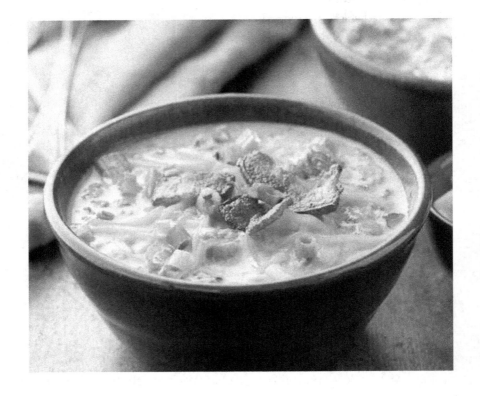

Lemony Chicken and Chive Soup

Preparation time: 10 minutes
Cooking time: 4 hours
Servings: 4

Ingredients:
2 boneless, skinless chicken breasts
6 cups chicken broth
¼ cup freshly squeezed lemon juice
2 tablespoons chives, chopped
yellow onion, chopped
cloves garlic, choppedSalt and pepper, to taste

Directions:
Add all the ingredients to a slow cooker and cook on high for 4 hours.
Once cooked, shred the chicken and stir back into the soup.

Nutrition:
calories 172, fat 5.9g, protein 22.1g, carbs 6.0g, net carbs 5.0g, fiber 1.0g

Chicken and Jalapeño Soup

Preparation time: 10 minutes
Cooking time: 4 hours
Servings: 6

Ingredients:
6 cups chicken broth
3 boneless, skinless chicken breasts
Juice from 1 lime
yellow onion, chopped
cloves garlic, chopped
1 jalapeño pepper, seeded and sliced
1 handful fresh cilantro
Salt and black pepper, to taste

Directions:
Add all the ingredients minus the cilantro, salt and black pepper to the base of a slow cooker and cook on high for 4 hours.
Add the cilantro and season with salt and black pepper.
Shred the chicken and serve.

Nutrition:
calories 110, fat 3.0g, protein 16.0g, carbs 4.0g, net carbs 3.0g, fiber 1.0g

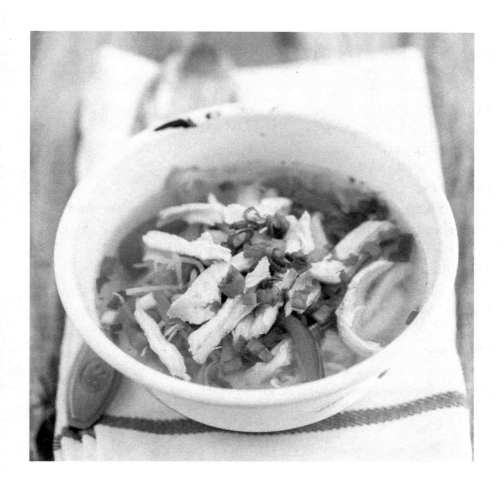

Butternut Squash Soup

Preparation time: 15 minutes
Cooking time: 7 hours
Servings: 5

Ingredients:
cups butternut squash, chopped
1 cup carrot, chopped
cups chicken stock
1 cup heavy cream
1 teaspoon ground cardamom
1 teaspoon ground cinnamon

Directions:
Put the butternut squash in the slow cooker. Sprinkle it with ground cardamom and ground cinnamon. Then add carrot and chicken stock. Close the lid and cook the soup on High for 5 hours.
Then blend the soup until smooth with the help of the immersion blender and add heavy cream.
Cook the soup on high for 2 hours more.

Nutrition:
125 calories, 1.7g protein,10.5g carbohydrates, 9.3g fat, 2g fiber, 33mg cholesterol, 485mg sodium, 301mg potassium.

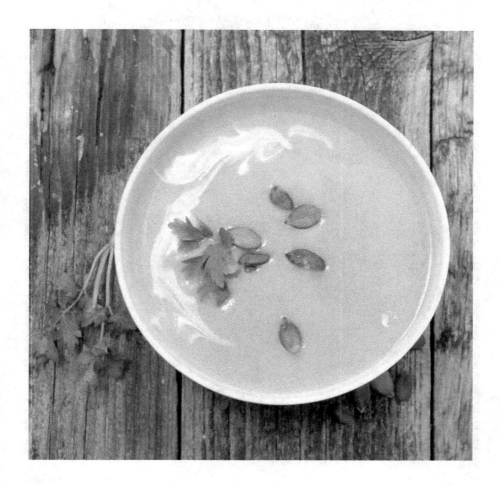

Snacks and Appetizer

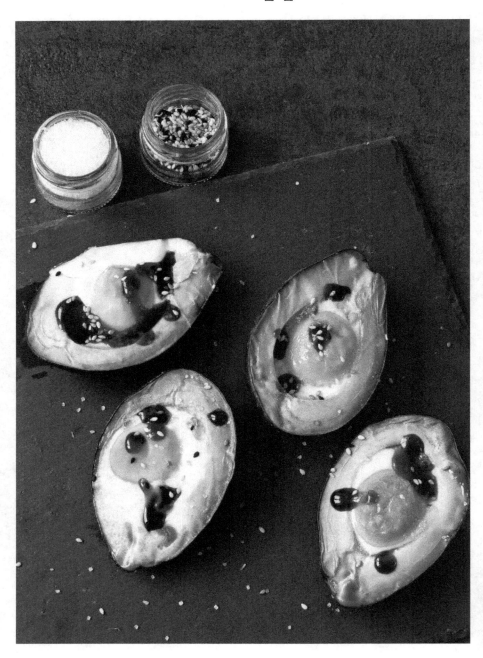

Bacon-Wrapped Poblano Poppers

Preparation time: 15 minutes
Cooking time: 30 minutes
Servings: 16

Ingredients:

10 ounces (283 g) cottage cheese, at room temperature
6 ounces (170 g) Swiss cheese, shredded
Sea salt and ground black pepper, to taste
½ teaspoon shallot powder
½ teaspoon cumin powder
⅓ teaspoon mustard seeds
16 poblano peppers, deveined and halved
16 thin slices bacon, sliced lengthwise

Directions:

Mix the cheese, salt, black pepper, shallot powder, cumin, and
mustard seeds until well combined.
Divide the mixture between the pepper halves. Wrap each pepper with 2 slices
of bacon; secure with toothpicks.
Arrange the stuffed peppers on the rack in the baking sheet.
Bake in the preheated oven at 390°F (199°C) for about 30 minutes until the
bacon is sizzling and browned. Bon appétit!

Nutrition:

calories 184, fat 14.1g, protein 8.9g, carbs 5.8g, net carbs 5.0g, fiber 0.8g

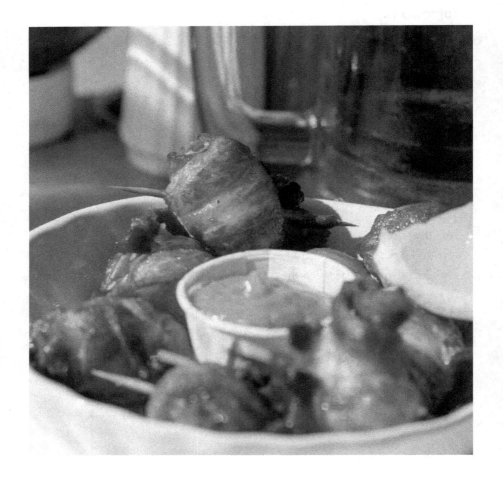

Artichoke and Spinach Dip

Preparation time: 10 minutes
Cooking time: 2 hours
Servings: 16

Ingredients:
(14-ounce) can artichoke hearts, drained and chopped
cups frozen chopped spinach, thawed and squeezed dry
1 tablespoon minced garlic
½ cup 2% milk
1 (8-ounce) package cream cheese, at room temperature
1 cup grated Parmesan cheese
¼ teaspoon sea salt
⅛ teaspoon freshly ground black pepper

Directions:
Place the artichoke hearts, spinach, garlic, milk, cream cheese,
Parmesan, salt, and pepper in a 2-quart slow cooker. Stir well to
combine.
Cover and cook on low for 2 hours, or until the cheese is melted and
the dip is hot.
Serve the dip in the slow cooker with the heat on low or "keep warm."

Nutrition:
calories 96, fat 7g, saturated fat 4g, cholesterol 21mg, carbohydrates 4g,
fiber 1g, protein 5g, sodium 278mg

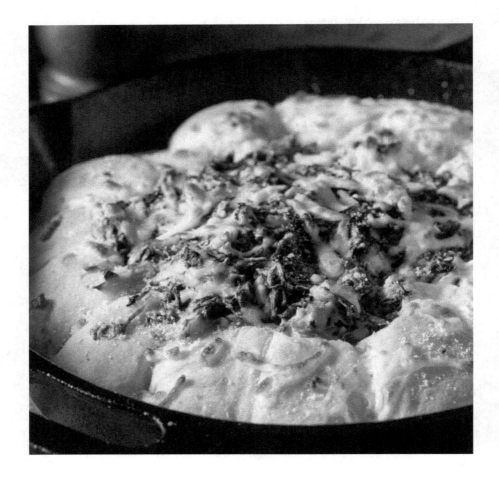

Mexican Chorizo and Squash Omelet

Preparation time: 10 minutes
Cooking time: 5 minutes
Servings: 4

Ingredients:

8 eggs, beaten
8 ounces (227 g) chorizo sausages, chopped
½ cup cotija cheese, crumbled
8 ounces (227 g) roasted squash, mashed
2 tablespoons olive oil
Salt and black pepper, to taste
Cilantro to garnish

Directions:

Season the eggs with salt and pepper and stir in the cotija cheese and squash. Heat half of olive oil in a pan over medium heat. Add chorizo sausage and cook until browned on all sides, turning occasionally. Drizzle the remaining olive oil and pour the egg mixture over.

Cook for 4 minutes until the eggs are cooked and lightly browned. Remove the pan and run a spatula around the edges of the omelet; slide onto a platter. Fold in half; serve sprinkled with cilantro.

Nutrition:

calories 684, fat 52.1g, protein 38.2g, carbs 9.3g, net carbs 8.4g, fiber 0.9g

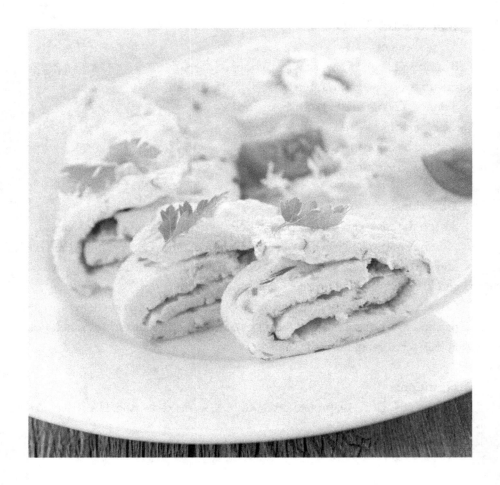

Stuffed Pepper s Platter

Preparation time: 10 minutes
Cooking time: 4 hours
Servings: 2

Ingredients:
red onion, chopped
1 teaspoons olive oil
½ teaspoon sweet paprika
½ tablespoon chili powder
1 garlic clove, minced
1 cup white rice, cooked
½ cup corn
A pinch of salt and black pepper
colored bell peppers, tops and insides scooped out
½ cup tomato sauce

Directions:
In a bowl, mix the onion with the oil, paprika and the other ingredients except the peppers and tomato sauce, stir well and stuff the peppers the with this mix.
Put the peppers in the slow cooker, add the sauce, put the lid on and cook on Low for 4 hours.
Transfer the peppers on a platter and serve as an appetizer.

Nutrition:
calories 253, fat 5g, fiber 4g, carbs 12g, protein 3g

Nacho Beans Dip

Preparation time: 10 minutes
Cooking time: 1 hour
Servings: 2

Ingredients:
¼ cup salsa
cup canned refried beans
½ cup nacho cheese
1 tablespoon green onions, chopped

Directions:
In your slow cooker, mix refried beans with salsa, nacho cheese and green onions, stir, cover and cook on High for 1 hour.
Divide into bowls and serve as a party dip Enjoy!

Nutrition:
calories 302, fat 5g, fiber 10g, carbs 16g, protein 6g

Deviled Eggs

Preparation time: 10 minutes
Cooking time: 20 minutes
Servings: 6

Ingredients:
6 eggs
1 tablespoon green tabasco
⅓ cup sugar-free mayonnaise

Directions:
Place the eggs in a saucepan, and cover with salted water. Bring to a boil over medium heat. Boil for 8 minutes. Place the eggs in an ice bath and let cool for 10 minutes. Peel and slice them in. Whisk together the tabasco, mayonnaise, and salt in a small bowl. Spoon this mixture on top of every egg.

Nutrition:
calories 180, fat 17.0g, protein 6.0g, carbs 5.0g, net carbs 5.0g, fiber 0g

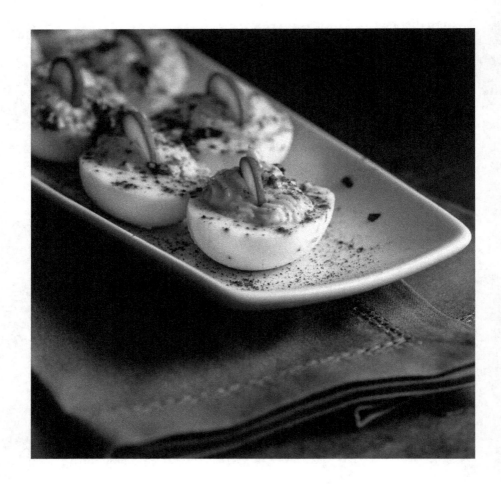

French Onion Dip

Preparation time: 15 minutes
Cooking time: 7 hours
Servings: 16

Ingredients:

4 yellow onions, thinly sliced
2 tablespoons extra-virgin olive oil
1 tablespoon unsalted butter
½ teaspoon sea salt
Pinch granulated sugar
½ cup sour cream
½ cup mayonnaise
⅛ teaspoon freshly ground black pepper

Directions:

Place the onions, olive oil, and butter in a 3-quart slow cooker. Season with the salt and sugar and stir to combine. Cover and cook on high for 6 to 8 hours, or until the onions are a rich, dark brown. If you're around during the day, stir the onions every 2 to 3 hours to prevent burning. .Transfer the cooked onions to a food processor using a slotted spoon. Process until still slightly chunky. Add the sour cream, mayonnaise, and pepper and pulse until thoroughly combined. Cover the dip and chill for 3 to 4 hours before serving. Refrigerate leftovers in an airtight container up to 4 days. This recipe does not freeze well.

Nutrition:

calories 95, fat 9g, saturated fat 3g, cholesterol 7mg, carbohydrates 3g, fiber 1g, protein 1g, sodium 112mg

Dessert

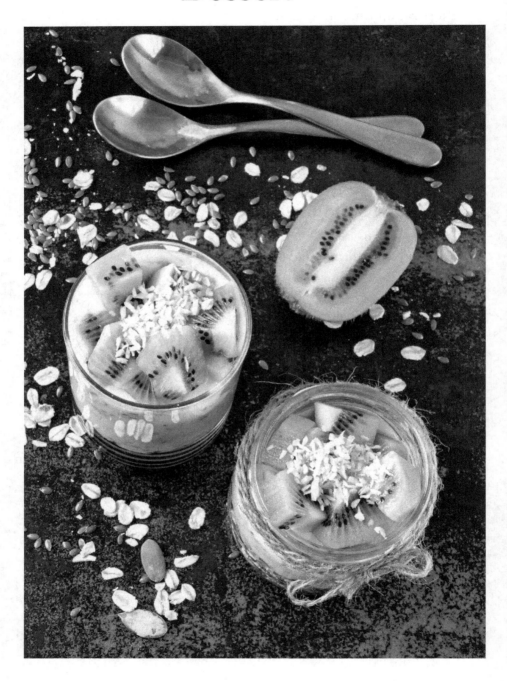

Coconut Chia Pudding

Preparation Time: 10 minutes
Cooking Time: 0 minutes
Servings: 1

Ingredients:
1/4 cup chia seeds
1/4 cup coconut milk
tbsp. unsweetened coconut
tsp. vanilla extract
tbsp. maple syrup

Directions:
Soak chia seeds in water for 2 to 3 minutes.

Take a bowl, add coconut milk, maple syrup, vanilla extract, and chia seeds and whisk them well.

Let it aside and mix again after 5 minutes.

Put it in an airtight bag and place it in the refrigerator for 1 hour. Serve and enjoy chilled coconut chia pudding.

Nutrition:
calories 165, fat 1.4g, fiber 5.4g, carbohydrates 1.2 g, protein 3.1g

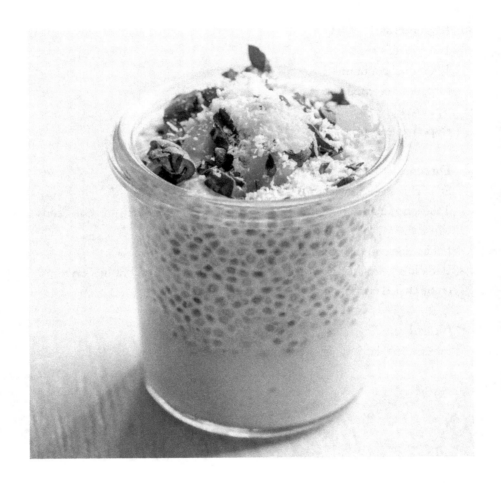

Apples with Raisins

Preparation time: 10 minutes
Cooking time: 5 hours
Servings: 4

Ingredients:
4 big apples
4 teaspoons raisins
4 teaspoons sugar
½ teaspoon ground cinnamon
½ cup of water

Directions:
Core the apples and fill them with sugar and raisins.
Then arrange the apples in the slow cooker.
Sprinkle them with ground cinnamon.
Add water and close the lid.
Cook the apples on low for 5 hours.

Nutrition:
141 calories, 0.7g protein,37.4g carbohydrates, 0.4g fat, 5.7g fiber,
0mg cholesterol, 3mg sodium, 263mg potassium.

Cream Mousse

Preparation time: 10 minutes
Cooking time: 0 minutes
Servings: 4

Ingredients:
2 cups double cream
4 egg yolks
½ teaspoon instant coffee
1 teaspoon pure coconut extract
6 tablespoons Xylitol

Directions:
Heat the cream in a pan over low heat; let it cool slightly.
Then, whisk the egg yolks with the instant coffee, coconut extract, and Xylitol until well combined.
Add the egg mixture to the lukewarm cream. Warm the mixture over low heat until it has reduced and thickened.
Refrigerate for 3 hours before serving. Enjoy!

Nutrition:
calories 290, fat 27.7g, protein 6.0g, carbs 5.0g, net carbs 5.0g, fiber 0g

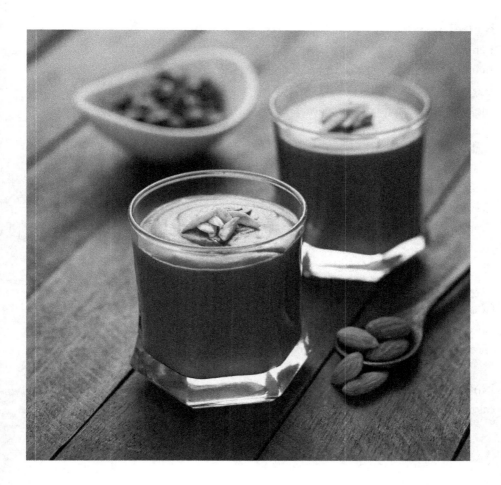

Tender Lime Cake

Preparation time: 20 minutes
Cooking time: 4 hours
Servings: 12

Ingredients:
1 lime, sliced
1 cup almond milk, unsweetened
1 ½ cup coconut flour
1 teaspoon vanilla extract
1 teaspoon baking powder
3 tablespoons Erythritol

Directions:
Combine the almond milk, coconut flour, vanilla extract, baking powder, and Erythritol.
Add the vanilla extract and stir until smooth.
Place the mixture in the slow cooker.
Then place the sliced lime over the cake.
Cook for 4 hours on High.
Check if the cake is cooked and chill.
Slice the cake into servings and enjoy!

Nutrition:
calories 109, fat 6.3g, fiber 6.6g, carbs 8g, protein 2.5g

Rum Brownies

Preparation time: 15 minutes
Cooking time: 22 minutes
Serving: 8

Ingredients:
⅔ cup almond flour
½ cup coconut flour
1 teaspoon baking powder
cup xylitol
½ cup cocoa powder, unsweetened
eggs
6 ounces (170 g) butter, melted
3 ounces (85 g) baking chocolate, unsweetened and melted
2 tablespoons rum
A pinch of salt
A pinch of freshly grated nutmeg
¼ teaspoon ground cinnamon

Directions:
In a mixing bowl, thoroughly combine dry ingredients. In a separate bowl, mix all the wet ingredients until well combined.
Stir dry mixture into wet ingredients. Evenly spread the batter into a parchment-lined baking dish.
Bake in the preheated oven at 360°F (182°C) for 20 to 22 minutes, until your brownies are set. Cut into squares and serve.

Nutrition:
calories 321, fat 30.1g, protein 5.7g, carbs 6.2g, net carbs 2.6g, fiber 3.6g

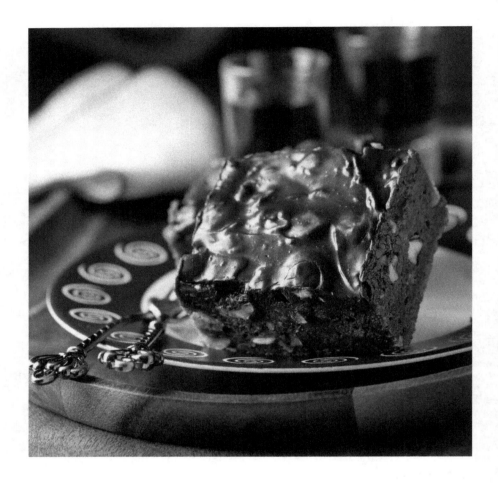

Panna Cotta

Preparation time: 10 minutes
Cooking time: 20 minutes
Servings: 4

Ingredients:

Unsalted butter, for greasing
tablespoons unflavored gelatin
tablespoons cold water
2 cups heavy whipping cream
⅓ cup granulated erythritol–monk fruit blend; less sweet: 3 tablespoons
½ teaspoon vanilla extract
½ teaspoon espresso instant powder
⅛ teaspoon salt

Directions:

Grease the silicone molds with butter and set aside.
In the small mixing bowl, dissolve the gelatin in the cold water and set aside.
In the medium saucepan, boil the heavy cream on medium heat. Lower the heat and simmer for about 4 minutes, until the cream begins to thicken.
Add the erythritol–monk fruit blend, vanilla, espresso powder, and salt.
Continue to stir to combine all the ingredients. Remove from the heat and add the dissolved gelatin. Stir until the gelatin is well incorporated.
Pour the mixture into the molds and allow it to cool at room temperature for about 30 minutes. After cooling, cover the molds with plastic wrap and put them in the refrigerator for at least 4 hours before taking the panna cotta out of the molds. Serve cold.
Store leftovers in an airtight container in the refrigerator for up to 3 days.

Nutrition:

calories 451, fat 46.8g, protein 6.0g, carbs 2.9g, net carbs 2.9g, fiber 0g

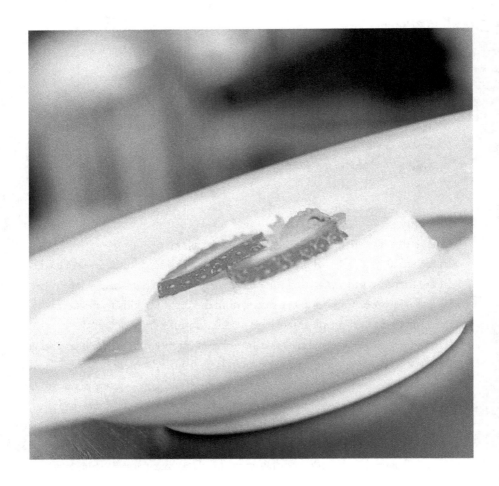

Tomato Jam

Preparation time: 10 minutes
Cooking time: 3 hours
Servings: 2

Ingredients
½ pound tomatoes, chopped
green apple, grated
tablespoons red wine vinegar
4 tablespoons sugar

Directions:
In your slow cooker, mix the tomatoes with the apple and the other ingredients, whisk, put the lid on and cook on Low for 3 hours.
Whisk the jam well, blend a bit using an immersion blender, divide into bowls and serve cold.

Nutrition:
calories 70, fat 1g, fiber 1g, carbs 18g, protein 1g

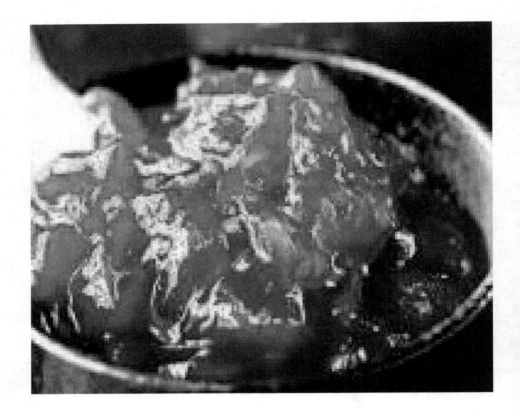

Other Keto Recipes

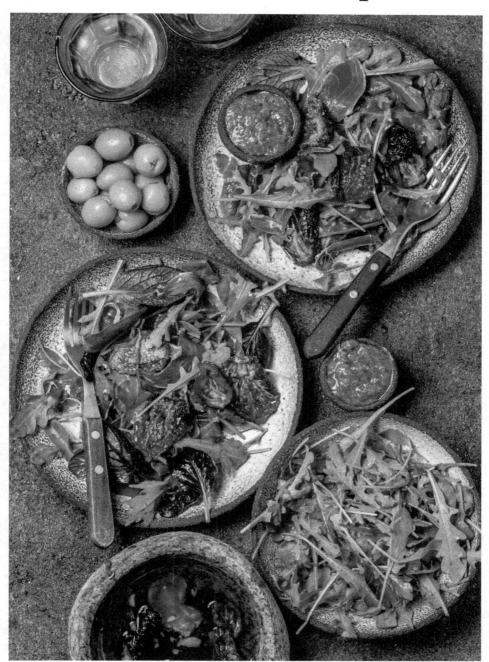

Pumpkin Bread

Preparation time: 10 minutes
Cooking time: 2 hours
Servings: 2

Ingredients:
Cooking spray
½ cup white flour
½ cup whole wheat flour
½ teaspoon baking soda
pinch of cinnamon powder
2 tablespoons olive oil
2 tablespoons maple syrup
2 egg
½ tablespoon milk
½ teaspoon vanilla extract
½ cup pumpkin puree
tablespoons walnuts, chopped
2 tablespoons chocolate chips

Directions:
In a bowl, mix white flour with whole wheat flour, baking soda and cinnamon and stir.
Add maple syrup, olive oil, egg, milk, vanilla extract, pumpkin puree, walnuts and chocolate chips and stir well.
Grease a loaf pan that fits your slow cooker with cooking spray, pour pumpkin bread, transfer to your cooker and cook on High for 2 hours.
Slice bread, divide between plates and serve.
Enjoy!

Nutrition:
calories 200, fat 3g, fiber 5g, carbs 8g, protein 4

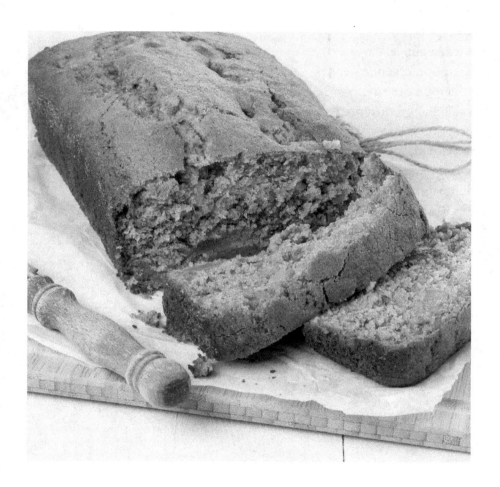

Stuffed Chicken

Preparation time: 15 minutes
Cooking time: 30 minutes
Servings: 5

Ingredients:
2 tablespoons olive oil
5 chicken cutlets
½ teaspoon cayenne pepper
½ teaspoon oregano
Sea salt and ground black pepper, to taste
tablespoon Dijon mustard
garlic cloves, minced
5 Italian peppers, deveined and chopped
1 chili pepper, chopped
1 cup Romano cheese, shredded
5 tablespoons sauerkraut, for serving

Directions:

Brush a baking pan with 1 tablespoon of the olive oil. Bruch the chicken cutlets with the remaining tablespoon of olive oil.

Season the chicken cutlets with the cayenne pepper, oregano, salt, and black pepper. Spread mustard on one side of each chicken cutlet.

Divide the garlic, peppers, and Romano cheese on the mustard side. Roll up tightly and use toothpicks to secure your rolls. Transfer to the prepared baking pan.

Bake in the preheated oven at 370°F (188°C) for about 30 minutes until golden brown on all sides (an instant-read thermometer should register 165°F (74°C)).

Spoon the sauerkraut over the chicken and serve. Bon appétit!

Nutrition:

calories 378, fat 16.6g, protein 47.0g, carbs 5.7g, net carbs 4.7g, fiber 1.0g

Pork with Cabbage

Preparation time: 15 minutes
Cooking time: 1 hour 15 minutes
Servings: 6

Ingredients:
2 tablespoons olive oil
2 pounds (907 g) pork stew meat, cubed
Salt and black pepper, to taste
2 tablespoons butter
4 garlic cloves, minced
¾ cup vegetable stock
½ cup white wine
3 carrots, chopped
1 cabbage head, shredded
½ cup scallions, chopped
1 cup heavy cream

Directions:
Set a pan over medium heat and warm butter and oil. Sear the pork
until brown. Add garlic, scallions and carrots; sauté for 5 minutes. Pour
in the cabbage, stock and wine, and bring to a boil. Reduce the heat
and cook for 1 hour covered. Add in heavy cream as you stir for 1
minute, adjust seasonings and serve.

Nutrition:
calories 512, fat 32.6g, protein 42.9g, carbs 9.3g, net carbs 5.9g,
fiber 3.4g

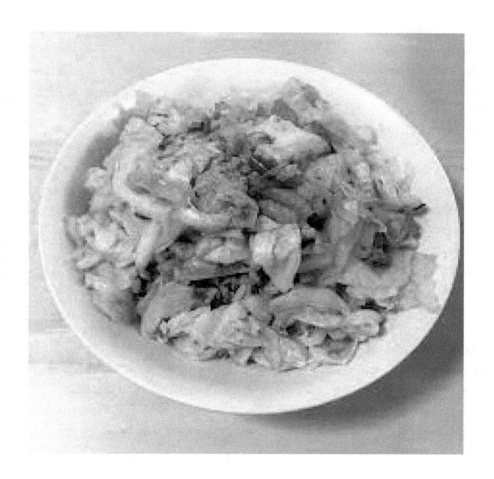

Beef with Mushrooms

Preparation time: 15 minutes
Cooking time: 3 hours 10 minutes
Servings: 6

Ingredients:
2 pounds (907 g) beef chuck roast, cubed
2 tablespoons olive oil
14.5 ounces (411 g) canned diced tomatoes
2 carrots, chopped
Salt and black pepper, to taste
½ pound (227 g) mushrooms, sliced
2 celery stalks, chopped
2 yellow onions, chopped
1 cup beef stock
1 tablespoon fresh thyme, chopped
½ teaspoon dry mustard
3 tablespoons almond flour

Directions:
Set an ovenproof pot over medium heat, warm olive oil and brown the beef on each side for a few minutes. Stir in the tomatoes, onions, salt, pepper, mustard, carrots, mushrooms, celery, and stock.
In a bowl, combine 1 cup water with flour. Place this to the pot, stir then set in the oven, and bake for 3 hours at 325°F (163°C) stirring at intervals of 30 minutes. Scatter the fresh thyme over and serve warm.

Nutrition:
calories 326, fat 18.1g, protein 28.1g, carbs 10.4g, net carbs 6.9g, fiber 3.5g

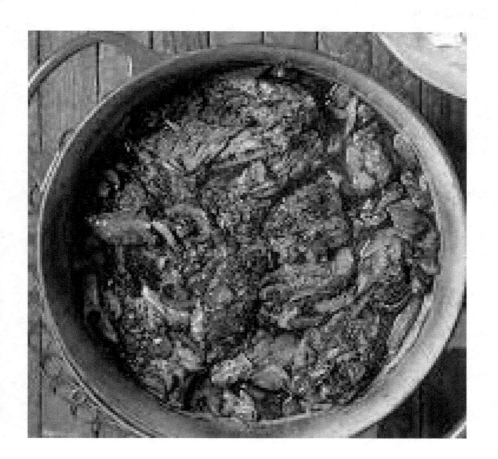

Crab Meatballs

Preparation time: 10 minutes
Cooking time: 5 minutes
Servings: 4

Ingredients:
1 tablespoon coconut oil
1 pound (454 g) lump crab meat
1 teaspoon Dijon mustard
1 egg
¼ cup mayonnaise
1 tablespoon coconut flour
1 tablespoon cilantro, chopped

Directions:
In a bowl, add crab meat, mustard, mayonnaise, coconut flour, egg, cilantro, salt, and pepper; mix to combine. Make patties out of the mixture. Melt coconut oil in a skillet over medium heat. Add crab patties and cook for 2-3 minutes per side. Remove to kitchen paper. Serve.

Nutrition:
calories 316, fat 24.3g, protein 15.2g, carbs 1.8g, net carb 1.5g, fiber 0.3g

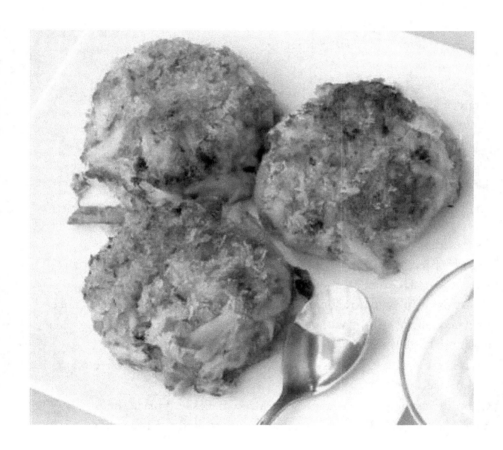

Roasted Asparagus and Tomatoes

Preparation time: 15 minutes
Cooking time: 20 minutes
Servings: 3

Ingredients:
1 pound (454 g) asparagus, trimmed
¼ teaspoon ground black pepper
Flaky salt, to season
3 tablespoons sesame seeds
1 tablespoon Dijon mustard
½ lime, freshly squeezed
3 tablespoons extra-virgin olive oil
2 garlic cloves, minced
1 tablespoon fresh tarragon, snipped
1 cup cherry tomatoes, sliced

Directions:
Start by preheating your oven to 400°F (205°C). Spritz a roasting pan with nonstick cooking spray.
Roast the asparagus for about 13 minutes, turning the spears over once or twice. Sprinkle with salt, pepper, and sesame seeds; roast an additional 3 to 4 minutes.
To make the dressing, whisk the Dijon mustard, lime juice, olive oil, and minced garlic.
Chop the asparagus spears into bite-sized pieces and place them in a nice salad bowl. Add the tarragon and tomatoes to the bowl; gently toss to combine.
Dress your salad and serve at room temperature. Enjoy!

Nutrition:
calories 160, fat 12.4g, protein 5.7g, carbs 6.2g, net carbs 2.2g, fiber 4.0

Cabbage Soup

Preparation Time: 10 minutes
Cooking Time: 30 minutes
Servings: 6

Ingredients:
1/4 cup onion, diced
1 clove garlic, minced
1 tsp. cumin
1 head cabbage, chopped
1 1/4 cup canned diced tomatoes
5 oz. canned green chilis
4 cups vegetable stock Salt and pepper to taste

Directions:
Heat a heavy stockpot over medium-high heat. Add the onions and sauté for 5- 7 minutes more. Add the garlic and sauté for one more minute.

Bring this in to a low simmer and cook until the vegetables are tender about 30 minutes. And add water, if necessary, during cooking.
Transfer to serving bowls and serve hot.

Nutrition:
calories 131, fat 4.3g, fiber 5.9g, carbohydrates 1.2g, protein 5.1g

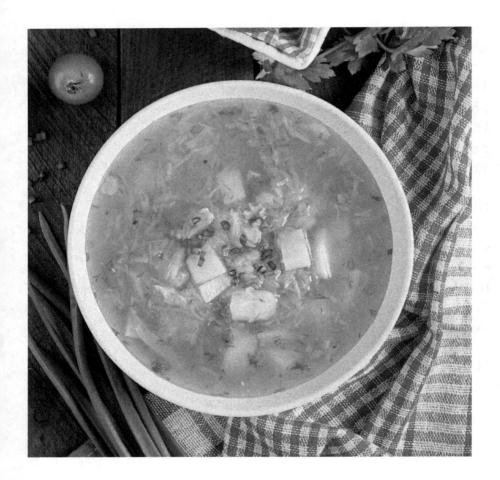

Spiced Chips with Cheese

Preparation Time: 15 minutes
Cooking Time: 15 minutes
Servings: 8

Ingredients:

3 tbsp. coconut flour
1/2 C. strong cheddar cheese, grated and divided
1/4 C. Parmesan cheese, grated
2 tbsp. butter, melted
1 organic egg
1 tsp. fresh thyme leaves, minced

Directions:

Preheat the oven to 3500 F. Line a large baking sheet with parchment paper.
In a bowl, place the coconut flour, 1/4 C. of grated cheddar, Parmesan, butter, and egg and mix until well combined.
Make eight equal-sized balls from the mixture.
Arrange the balls onto a prepared baking sheet in a single layer about 2-inch apart.
Form into flat discs.
Sprinkle each disc with the remaining cheddar, followed by thyme.
Bake for around 15 minutes.

Nutrition:

calories 101, fat 6.5g, fiber 1.4g, carbohydrates 1.2g, protein 3.1g

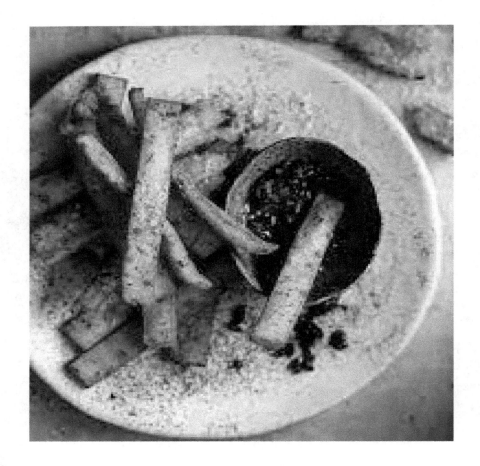

Dark Chocolate

Preparation time: 10 minutes
Cooking time: 0 minutes
Makes: 15 pieces

Ingredients:

¾ cup coconut oil
¼ cup confectioners' erythritol–monk fruit blend; less sweet: 3 tablespoons
3 tablespoons dark cocoa powder
½ cup slivered almonds
¾ teaspoon almond extract

Directions:

Line the baking pan with parchment paper and set aside.

In the microwave-safe bowl, melt the coconut oil in the microwave in 10-second intervals.

In the medium bowl, whisk together the melted coconut oil, confectioners' erythritol–monk fruit blend, and cocoa powder until fully combined. Stir in the slivered almonds and almond extract.

Pour the mixture into the prepared baking pan and spread evenly. Put the pan in the freezer for about 20 minutes, or until the chocolate bark is solid.

Once the chocolate bark is solid, break apart into 15 roughly even pieces to serve.

Store the chocolate bark in an airtight container in the freezer. Allow to slightly thaw about 5 minutes before eating. Thaw only what you will be eating.

Nutrition:

calories 118, fat 13.0g, protein 1.0g, carb 1.0g, net carbs 0g, fiber 1g

Raspberry Tart

Preparating time: 20 minutes
Cooking tima: 4 hours
Servings: 6

Ingredients:
1 cup raspberries
4 tablespoons coconut flour
4 tablespoons butter
3 tablespoons Erythritol
1 teaspoon vanilla extract
1 teaspoon ground ginger

Directions:
Combine butter, coconut flour, ground ginger, and vanilla extract.
Knead the dough.
Cover the bottom of the slow cooker with parchment.
Place the dough in the slow cooker and flatten it to the shape of a pie crust.
Place the raspberries over the piecrust and sprinkle with Erythritol.
Cook the tart for 4 hours on High.
Serve the cooked tart chilled.

Nutrition:
calories 101, fat 7.9g, fiber 1.5g, carbs 14.2g, protein 0.9g

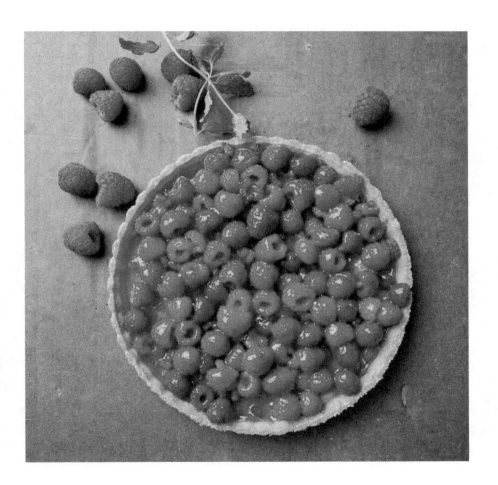